COMPLETE GUIDE TO HEMORRHOIDECTOMY

Comprehensive Handbook To Surgical Treatment, Recovery, Pain Management, And Post Operative Care

DR. BRUNO HORAN

Copyright © 2023 by Dr. Bruno Horan

All rights reserved. Except for brief quotations embodied in critical reviews and certain other noncommercial uses permitted by copyright law, no part of this publication may be reproduced, distributed, or transmitted in any form or by any means, Including photocopying, recording, or other electronic or mechanical methods, without the prior written permission of the publisher.

Disclaimer:

The information provided in this book, is intended for general informational purposes only and should not be considered as professional advice.

The author has made every effort to ensure the accuracy of the information presented. However, readers are advised to consult with a qualified healthcare professional before attempting any herbal remedies or making significant changes to their wellness routine. Individual health conditions vary, and what may be suitable for one person may not be appropriate for another.

It is important to note that the author is not in any endorsement deal, partnership, or affiliation with any organization, brand, or company mentioned in this book. Any references to specific products or services are based on the author's personal experience or general knowledge and do not imply an endorsement or promotion of those products or services

Contents

CHAPTER ONE 21
PRE-OPERATIVE EVALUATION 21
Initial Consultation And Review Of Medical Records 21

Physical Assessment And Diagnostic Procedures . 22

Assessing Surgical Eligibility 23

Talking With Patients About The Benefits And Risks 24

Process Of Informed Consent 25

CHAPTER TWO 27
HEMORROWIDECTOMY TYPES 27
Conventional Hemorrhoidectomy (Excisional) 27

Surgical Hemorrhage 28

Rubber Band Ligation 30

Hemorrhoidectomy Using Laser 31

Comparing Different Methods 32

CHAPTER THREE 35
SURGICAL MANAGEMENT 35
Comprehensive Procedure For A Conventional Hemorrhoidectomy 35

Options And Considerations For Anesthesia 36
Materials And Instruments Used In Surgery 38
Methods To Reduce Blood Loss And Infection 39

CHAPTER FOUR 43
REPAY AND RESUMMATION 43
Hospitalized Immediate Post-Operative Care 43
Pain Control With Drugs 44
Dietary And Lifestyle Modifications For Healing ... 45
Guidelines And Restrictions For Physical Activity . 48

CHAPTER FIVE 51
MANAGING COMPLICATIONS 51
Signs Of Infection And Preventive Actions 53
Managing Hemorrhage Following Surgery 54
Managing The Retention Of Urine 55
Long-Term Issues And Their Resolutions 56

CHAPTER SIX 59
END RESULTS AND POST-ITEMS 59
Keeping An Eye Out For Hemorrhoids To Recur .. 59
Long-Term Modifications To Lifestyle To Avoid
Recurrence 60
Frequent Follow-Up Plans 61

- Effect On Life Quality 62
- Case Studies And Patient Testimonials 63

CHAPTER SEVEN 65

HEMORRHOID TREATMENTS WITH ANOTHER APPROACH 65

- Synopsis Of Non-Surgical Interventions 65
- The Efficacy Of Dietary And Lifestyle Modifications 66
- Taking Over-The-Counter Drugs 67
- The Function Of Complementary And Alternative Medicine 68
- Comparative Analysis Of Surgical Results 69

CHAPTER EIGHT 73

FAQS & FREQUENTLY ASKED QUESTIONS 73

- Taking Care Of Common Patient Myths And Fears 73
- Expectations For Pain And Recovery Time 74
- Surgical Risks And Their Management 75
- Cost And Insurance Considerations 77
- Comprehensive Responses To Commonly Asked Questions 78

CONCERNING THIS BOOK

A thorough manual that explores all of the important facets of hemorrhoidectomy, "Hemorrhoidectomy" is a priceless resource for patients and medical professionals alike. A comprehensive introduction is provided in the first section, which also defines the different surgical techniques now in use and traces the historical development of hemorrhoidectomy treatments. This historical viewpoint not only draws attention to the improvements in medical science but also lays the groundwork for comprehending the standards and patient profiles that influence the choice to undergo surgery. The effectiveness and applicability of hemorrhoidectomy in contemporary medical practice are further highlighted by statistical insights into patient outcomes and success rates.

The steps needed in assessing a patient for surgery are carefully laid out in the pre-operative assessment part of the book. Comprehensive pre-operative evaluation is emphasized in this area, starting with the initial consultation and reviewing medical history, and continuing with physical examinations and diagnostic tests. The discourse continues with important talks about the advantages and disadvantages of the procedure, making sure patients are fully informed by way of a thorough informed consent procedure. This all-encompassing strategy guarantees that patients and medical professionals are ready for the upcoming surgical procedure.

The book explores the different methods of hemorrhoidectomy and offers a detailed comparison of techniques such as rubber band ligation, laser hemorrhoidectomy, stapled hemorrhoidopexy, and classic excisional hemorrhoidectomy. The in-depth explanation of each technique provides readers with a thorough knowledge of the procedural subtleties, benefits, and potential downsides. By helping medical practitioners choose the best approach for their patients, this comparative study improves surgical results and patient happiness.

The surgical technique section, which covers each stage of a conventional hemorrhoidectomy, is quite informative. This covers the many forms of anesthesia, the surgical tools and supplies, and methods to reduce bleeding and infection. Along with covering closure techniques and post-operative dressing, the book offers a comprehensive surgical roadmap that can be a great resource for medical professionals.

The book goes into great detail on two important phases: recovery and post-operative care. A thorough discussion is held regarding the guidelines for immediate care, pain management techniques, and necessary food and lifestyle changes. A comfortable recovery for patients is ensured by recommendations for physical activity limits and tips for managing common post-surgical symptoms. This emphasizes the significance of thorough post-operative care in attaining optimal surgical outcomes.

Another important topic covered in the book is managing complications, which includes doable fixes for typical post-operative problems like infections, bleeding, and urine retention. To ensure that healthcare professionals are prepared to face any difficulties that may develop during the healing process, it also addresses long-term consequences and associated treatments.

The significance of keeping an eye out for recurrence and making lifestyle modifications to avoid it is emphasized in the section on long-term outcomes and follow-up. The impact of regular follow-up programs on quality of life is discussed in depth, along with case studies and patient testimonies that offer practical insights into the long-term success of hemorrhoidectomy.

The book offers a summary of non-surgical choices for individuals who are thinking about them. It assesses the efficacy of over-the-counter drugs, herbal medicines, and dietary and lifestyle modifications. This balanced perspective provided by the comparison with surgical outcomes aids in the decision-making process for patients and healthcare professionals regarding the most appropriate course of action.

The book also tackles patient worries and myths, recovery expectations, hazards, and insurance considerations. Lastly, it answers frequently asked questions and concerns. This section guarantees that all possible questions are addressed in detail, giving patients thinking about a hemorrhoidectomy peace of mind and clarity. "Hemorrhoidectomy" is a valuable resource that walks readers through every facet of this common yet intricate surgical treatment with its comprehensive and interesting information.

Overview of Hemorrhoidectomy

Definition and Background Information

Hemorrhoids are enlarged veins in the lower rectum or anus that can be surgically removed. This treatment is known as a hemorrhoidectomy. Both internal and external hemorrhoids are possible, and they frequently result in pain, bleeding, and itching. The Greek terms "hemorrhoids" (vein likely to bleed) and "ektomď" (excision) are the source of the name "hemorrhoidectomy." Hippocrates' writings contain some of the earliest recorded accounts of the practice. The methods have changed dramatically throughout the years, with current approaches emphasizing the reduction of discomfort and healing time.

Various Hemorrhoidectomy Procedure Types

Hemorrhoidectomy operations come in a variety of forms, each customized to meet the unique requirements and medical circumstances of the patient. The most typical kinds consist of:

Excisional Hemorrhoidectomy: In this conventional technique, the hemorrhoidal tissue is surgically removed with a knife, scissors, or laser. In severe cases, it is very effective, although the recovery time is prolonged.

Stapled Hemorrhoidopexy (PPH): This technique involves removing a ring of extra tissue from the anal canal using a circular stapling device. By doing this, the hemorrhoid shrinks and the residual tissue is drawn back into place. Compared to the excisional procedure, it usually causes less discomfort and requires a shorter recovery period.

Hemorrhoidal Artery Ligation (HAL): Alternatively called transanal hemorrhoidal dearterialization (THD), this technique entails identifying the arteries supplying the hemorrhoids with a Doppler ultrasound and tying them off. As a result, the hemorrhoids receive less blood flow and eventually get smaller. It requires less time to recuperate from and is less intrusive.

Laser Hemorrhoidectomy: Hemorrhoidal tissue is removed using laser radiation. Compared to conventional surgical techniques, it results in less bleeding, less discomfort, and a quicker recovery period.

Selection Criteria for Surgery

The decision to operate on hemorrhoids is usually based on several variables, such as the patient's general health, the effectiveness of non-surgical treatments, and the severity of the symptoms. Hemorrhoidectomy eligibility requirements include:

The severity of Symptoms: If there is severe bleeding or discomfort that interferes with everyday activities, surgery is typically advised for third- and fourth-degree (permanently prolapsed) hemorrhoids.

Failure of Conservative Treatments: Surgery may be the next course of action if food, lifestyle, and pharmaceutical adjustments (such as topical creams and suppositories) do not result in relief.

Complications: Surgical surgery may be required in cases of thrombosed hemorrhoids (blood clots within hemorrhoids), recurring infections, or non-healing fissures.

Patient Preference and Lifestyle: Patients may opt for surgery if they would rather have a definitive therapy than continue with conservative management or if their lifestyle is greatly affected by hemorrhoid symptoms.

General Health: Before surgery, patients must be in good general health. Certain conditions, such as coagulopathy or serious cardiovascular disease, may call for extra care or different therapies.

Statistics and Patient Demographics

Adults between the ages of 45 and 65 are most frequently candidates for hemorrhoidectomy, while surgery can be required at any age in certain situations. According to statistics,

Gender Distribution: Although hemorrhoids can affect both men and women, some research indicates that women are slightly more likely to get them than men, especially during pregnancy and the postpartum period.

Prevalence: Hemorrhoids are thought to affect approximately 75% of people at some point in their lives; fewer people will need surgery to treat them.

Geographic and Lifestyle Factors: Hemorrhoidectomy incidence rates can differ depending on the area and way of living. Sedentary lifestyles, obesity, and low-fiber diets are important risk factors that lead to hemorrhoid development.

Healthcare Access: The frequency of hemorrhoidectomy procedures in various populations might be influenced by factors such as the availability of experienced surgeons and access to healthcare.

Overall Results and Success Ratios

After a hemorrhoidectomy, most patients get great symptom reduction and a high success rate. Important results and success rates consist of:

After surgery, more than 90% of patients report considerable improvement in their hemorrhoid symptoms, such as less pain, bleeding, and itching.

Recurrence Rates: Hemorrhoidectomy provides long-term relief, but there is a tiny possibility of recurrence, which can range from 5% to 10% based on the surgical technique and the patient's compliance with post-surgery lifestyle advice.

Complications: Pain, hemorrhage, infection, and retention of urine are possible side effects.

Improvements in surgical methods have reduced these dangers, nevertheless.

Recovery Time: Recovery timeframes might differ. For example, a typical excisional hemorrhoidectomy takes 2-4 weeks to heal, whereas less invasive procedures like stapled hemorrhoidopexy or HAL may allow patients to resume regular activities in as little as a week.

Patients can make educated decisions regarding their treatment options and expectations by being aware of the various types of hemorrhoidectomy procedures, surgical criteria, patient demographics, and general outcomes.

CHAPTER ONE

PRE-OPERATIVE EVALUATION

Initial Consultation And Review Of Medical Records

Consultation with a healthcare provider is the first stage in the pre-operative evaluation for a hemorrhoidectomy.

In this appointment, the doctor will collect a complete medical history. This includes finding out about the patient's history of bleeding disorders, current medical condition, and length of bleeding episodes.

Any underlying medical issues, such as diabetes, hypertension, or bleeding problems, will also be discussed with the patient's doctor because they may have an impact on the procedure and the healing period.

The doctor will also go over the patient's existing medications, including over-the-counter meds and vitamins, to look for any that might interact with anesthetic or post-operative prescriptions.

Physical Assessment And Diagnostic Procedures

To determine the extent of the hemorrhoids, a physical examination is conducted after the initial appointment.

Usually, this entails a visual assessment as well as a digital rectal examination to look for hemorrhoids and other possible problems like cracks or abscesses.

The physician may occasionally suggest further testing, such as a colonoscopy or sigmoidoscopy. By giving a more thorough picture of the colon and rectum, these tests aid in ruling out other illnesses that could cause symptoms similar to hemorrhoids.

To rule out anemia, infection, or other issues that can make surgery more difficult, blood tests may also be required.

Assessing Surgical Eligibility

Not every hemorrhoid patient will be a good candidate for surgery. To determine eligibility, the healthcare professional will assess the patient's general health, the severity of the hemorrhoids, and the efficacy of prior therapies.

A patient's age, way of life, and capacity for recuperation following surgery are among the variables taken into account.

Mildly symptomatic patients might be encouraged to stick with conservative measures including dietary adjustments, prescription drugs, or non-surgical procedures.

Patients with severe, ongoing problems that substantially affect their quality of life are usually advised to have surgery.

Talking With Patients About The Benefits And Risks

Before undergoing surgery, patients must have a thorough understanding of the advantages and possible hazards associated with hemorrhoidectomy.

The surgeon will go over the procedure, what to anticipate in the postoperative period and any possible issues. Pain, bleeding, infection, and problems with bowel motions after surgery are common hazards.

For those with severe symptoms, however, the advantages frequently exceed the risks and result in notable relief and an increase in quality of life.

The possibility of a hemorrhoid recurrence and the significance of lifestyle modifications to avoid complications in the future will also be discussed by the doctor.

Process Of Informed Consent

Obtaining informed permission is an essential step in getting ready for a hemorrhoidectomy. The medical professional will make sure the patient is completely aware of the procedure's goals, advantages, dangers, and available options.

The patient will be able to voice any concerns and ask questions. The patient will sign a consent document attesting to their understanding and approval of the surgery's continuation after they feel sufficiently informed.

This phase is crucial to ensure that the patient makes an informed healthcare decision on both ethical and legal grounds.

Healthcare professionals can assist in guaranteeing that patients are well-prepared for hemorrhoidectomy, resulting in better outcomes and a more seamless recovery process, by carefully attending to every facet of the pre-operative assessment.

CHAPTER TWO

HEMORROWIDECTOMY TYPES

The surgical operation known as a hemorrhoidectomy is used to remove hemorrhoids, which are enlarged and irritated veins in the rectum and anus that produce pain and bleeding. Hemorrhoidectomy can be done in several ways, each with a special method and advantages.

Conventional Hemorrhoidectomy (Excisional)

The most popular and thorough form of hemorrhoid removal is traditional excisional hemorrhoidectomy. Hemorrhoidal tissues are completely surgically excised during this surgery.

The patient is usually given either a regional or general anesthetic for the procedure. The hemorrhoid is incised around, and the enlarged veins are removed by the surgeon. After that, the wounds are either sutured shut or allowed to heal naturally. When it comes to treating large or severely prolapsed hemorrhoids, this treatment works quite well.

Because the anal region is sensitive, patients who have conventional hemorrhoidectomy frequently endure substantial pain throughout the postoperative period.

Effective pain management typically entails prescription drugs, sitz baths, and occasionally topical therapies.

This surgery has a high success rate and offers long-term relief from hemorrhoidal symptoms, despite the discomfort.

Surgical Hemorrhage

The Procedure for Prolapse and Hemorrhoids (PPH), commonly known as stapled hemorrhoidopexy, is a less invasive option than the conventional excisional procedure.

This method is placing the hemorrhoidal tissue back into the anal canal and fastening it with a circular stapling device, as opposed to eliminating the hemorrhoids.

By lowering the blood supply to the hemorrhoids, this technique causes them to contract and finally fall out. Usually, regional or general anesthesia is used during stapled hemorrhoidopexy.

Since the stapling is done above the anal canal's pain threshold, this procedure has several benefits over typical excisional hemorrhoidectomy, chief among them being a decrease in postoperative pain.

Patients usually recover more quickly and can resume their regular routines sooner. Stapled hemorrhoidopexy does provide a little increased risk of consequences, including anal stenosis and bleeding.

Rubber Band Ligation

Internal hemorrhoids can be treated with a minimally invasive treatment called rubber band ligation. This method entails severing the hemorrhoid's blood supply by wrapping a tiny rubber band around its base.

Anesthesia is not normally required for the procedure, which is performed in a physician's office. The doctor applies one or two small rubber bands tightly around the hemorrhoid using a device known as a ligator. Within a few days, the hemorrhoid shrivels up and falls out, generally with a bowel movement.

Smaller internal hemorrhoids can be successfully treated with rubber band ligation, which causes very little discomfort. A few days after the procedure, some patients may have slight pain or a sense of fullness in the rectum. With this approach, patients can almost immediately return to their regular activities and the success rate is high.

Hemorrhoidectomy Using Laser

Using laser technology, a contemporary method for hemorrhoid removal is called laser hemorrhoidectomy. This method entails slicing through the hemorrhoidal tissue with a concentrated laser beam.

Because of the laser's high degree of precision and precision, less damage is done to the surrounding tissues. Anesthesia of the local, regional, or general kind may be used for the procedure.

Compared to traditional procedures, laser hemorrhoidectomy frequently leads to less postoperative pain, decreased bleeding, and a quicker recovery.

Less tissue stress and smaller incisions assist patients by reducing the risk of infection and speeding up the healing process. Nevertheless, a laser hemorrhoidectomy may incur additional costs, and not all insurance policies may cover it.

Comparing Different Methods

Several variables are taken into consideration while comparing the various methods of hemorrhoidectomy, such as the extent of the hemorrhoids, the patient's choice, the length of recuperation, and any possible problems.

Conventional Hemorrhoidectomy with Excision:

Advantages: Provides long-lasting relief from big, prolapsed hemorrhoids.

Cons: Prolonged recovery period and severe postoperative discomfort.

The stapled hemorrhoidectomy

Benefits: Faster healing and less discomfort following surgery.

Cons: There is a little increased chance of problems and recurrence.

Rubber Band Ligation:

Positives: Fast recovery; little discomfort; minimum invasiveness.

Cons: May need more than one treatment; best for tiny internal hemorrhoids.

Hemorrhoidectomy with laser:

Advantages: Faster healing; accuracy; less discomfort and bleeding.

Cons: More expensive; limited availability.

Depending on the patient's preferences and particular condition, each technique has unique benefits and may be more appropriate for some patients than others. You must speak with a healthcare professional to ascertain the best course of action given your unique situation.

CHAPTER THREE
SURGICAL MANAGEMENT

Comprehensive Procedure For A Conventional Hemorrhoidectomy

The goal of a typical hemorrhoidectomy is to remove large, bothersome hemorrhoids surgically. To allow for the best possible access to the surgical site, the patient is first positioned, usually in the lithotomy or prone position. After that, the surgical site is meticulously cleaned and ready.

Little incisions are made by the surgeon all around the hemorrhoid tissue. The judicious placement of these incisions is intended to limit harm to the surrounding healthy tissue.

Using precise dissection procedures, the hemorrhoid is gently detached from the underlying muscle so that the blood vessels supplying the hemorrhoid can be identified and controlled properly.

Following the excision of the hemorrhoid, any bleeding arteries are tied up.

With great care, the entire hemorrhoidal tissue is excised in an attempt to avoid recurrence, while also preserving as much healthy rectal and anal canal tissue as feasible.

The surgeon carefully examines the region after removing the hemorrhoids to make sure all troublesome tissue has been removed and to stop any bleeding that may have remained.

Options And Considerations For Anesthesia

For a hemorrhoidectomy, there are various anesthetic choices, each with unique advantages and drawbacks. The patient's health, preferences, and the surgeon's advice all play a role in the anesthetic choice.

Local anesthesia entails numbing just the surgical site, so the patient can undergo the treatment while awake and pain-free. To aid in the patient's relaxation, sedation is frequently added to it.

Regional anesthesia refers to the process of numbing the lower body by injecting an anesthetic close to the spinal cord, also known as spinal or epidural anesthesia. It lets the sufferer stay awake and offers great pain relief.

General anesthesia: This technique induces a deep sleep in the patient, guaranteeing that they are pain-free and unconscious throughout the procedure. When a patient wishes to remain unconscious or for more involved operations, general anesthesia is usually utilized.

To protect patient safety and comfort, particular preoperative and postoperative measures are needed for each type of anesthesia. To assist the patient in making an informed choice, the anesthesiologist will go over the advantages and disadvantages of each alternative.

Materials And Instruments Used In Surgery

The accuracy and potency of the surgical tools and supplies utilized during a hemorrhoidectomy determine its outcome. Typical instruments consist of:

A scalpel is used to carefully cut the tissue surrounding the hemorrhage.

Hemostats: Instruments for clamping blood vessels during a process.

Scissors: For cutting stitches and tissue.

An instrument that reduces bleeding by cauterizing blood vessels with electrical currents is called an electrocautery device.

Threads used to seal incisions and tie off blood vessels are called sutures and ligatures.

To maintain improved visualization and keep the surgery area open, specific retractors may also be utilized. To reduce the danger of infection both before and after the surgery, sterile dressings and antiseptic solutions are crucial.

Methods To Reduce Blood Loss And Infection

A good hemorrhoidectomy and a speedy recovery depend on minimizing bleeding and infection. Surgeons use a variety of methods to do this:

Meticulous Hemostasis: During surgery, bleeding should be meticulously controlled using hemostats and electrocautery equipment.

Antiseptic Protocols: To avoid bacterial contamination, the surgical site should be thoroughly cleaned, and sterile tools should be used.

The use of antibiotics both before and after surgery to lower the risk of infection is known as antibiotic prophylaxis.

Gentle Tissue Handling: This technique can lessen postoperative bleeding and inflammation by avoiding using undue force or stress on the surrounding tissues.

These methods aid in ensuring patient safety and fostering the best possible healing when paired with meticulous surgical planning and execution.

Closure Techniques and Dressing After Surgery

To promote healing and avoid problems, the surgical site must be appropriately closed and treated following the hemorrhoidectomy. Depending on the particular instance and the surgeon's preference, many closure techniques are used:

Primary Closure: After the hemorrhoid is removed, the incisions are sutured. This approach lowers the chance of infection and encourages quicker healing.

Open Technique: In some circumstances, leaving the incision open to heal secondary purposes might lessen postoperative pain and complications.

Stapled Hemorrhoidectomy: This technique, which frequently reduces postoperative pain, involves removing and closing the hemorrhoid tissue in a single phase using a circular stapling device.

Applying sterile gauze and absorbent pads to the surgical site is known as post-operative dressing. These dressings lessen the chance of infection, shield the incision, and absorb any drainage.

The patient receives instructions on wound care, including dressing changes and keeping an eye out for signs of infection or heavy bleeding.

In summary, careful attention to closure techniques and appropriate postoperative care are critical for a speedy recovery and reduction of problems after a hemorrhoidectomy.

CHAPTER FOUR

REPAY AND RESUMMATION

Hospitalized Immediate Post-Operative Care

You will be closely watched in the hospital following a hemorrhoidectomy to make sure your recovery from the procedure goes well. Your blood pressure, heart rate, and oxygen saturation will all be regularly checked. This time is critical for taking care of any urgent issues and making sure you're comfortable.

Following the procedure, you should anticipate some discomfort and possibly pain. Medication for pain will be administered as needed by physicians and nurses. If drainage tubes were inserted during the treatment, they might also provide you with instructions on how to take care of them and change dressings. When you can begin drinking fluids and following a light diet will be decided by your doctor.

It's critical that you carefully adhere to your healthcare team's advice throughout this early phase of rehabilitation. To minimize tension on the surgery site, this entails remaining in bed or moving around only as directed. To lower your risk of issues like blood clots, nurses may advise you on how to position yourself properly and may even push for early ambulation.

Pain Control With Drugs

One of the most important aspects of recuperating after a hemorrhoidectomy is pain management. You will probably be given oral or IV pain medication right after the surgery. The intention is to minimize adverse effects while maintaining your comfort. Depending on your unique needs and response, your healthcare team will modify the kind and dosage of pain medication you use.

Your physician will write prescriptions for painkillers that you can take as needed when you go from hospital care to at-home care. These could include prescription opioids for more severe pain or over-the-counter drugs like acetaminophen. It's vital to follow the dose recommendations attentively and to not exceed the suggested amounts to avoid issues.

Your doctor could suggest sitz baths or cold packs in addition to prescription drugs for pain relief. These can help minimize swelling and discomfort around the surgery site. You must let your medical team know if there are any changes in your symptoms or pain so they can modify your treatment strategy.

Dietary And Lifestyle Modifications For Healing

Your food and way of living may need to change temporarily following a hemorrhoidectomy to aid in healing and minimize discomfort. You may begin with a clear liquid diet at first and work your way up to solid foods as you are able. Constipation can put a strain on the surgical area, therefore it's critical to avoid it and drink enough water.

You may receive particular food instructions to adhere to during your recuperation from your physician or a nutritionist.

To encourage regular bowel movements, you could try increasing the amount of fruits, vegetables, and whole grains in your meals. In the early phases of recuperation, avoiding alcohol and spicy foods can also help prevent discomfort.

You might need to temporarily give up physically demanding tasks like heavy lifting or vigorous exercise. Depending on how well you are recovering, your doctor will advise you on when to get back to your regular activities.

Without putting undue stress on the surgical site, taking quick walks and doing light stretches will assist enhance circulation and encourage recovery.

Some Advice for Handling Typical Post-Surgical Symptoms

You can have typical post-hemorrhoidectomy symptoms including light bleeding, itching, or discomfort throughout the healing phase. Although these symptoms usually go better as the surgical site heals, you can control them nonetheless:

Light bleeding following surgery is common. You could be told not to strain when having a bowel movement and to use sanitary pads instead of tampons.

Itching: Reducing itching can be achieved by keeping the anal region dry and clean. For comfort, your doctor could suggest taking a sitz bath or using soft, fragrance-free wipes.

Pain: Using cold packs on the affected area and taking over-the-counter painkillers can help control pain. Steer clear of prolonged sitting and think about using a pillow or cushion for extra support.

It's critical to communicate any worries or newly noticed symptoms as soon as possible with your healthcare professional. They can offer tailored advice to meet your unique requirements and guarantee a speedy recovery.

Guidelines And Restrictions For Physical Activity

Your doctor will give you precise instructions on physical activity after a hemorrhoidectomy to promote recovery and avoid problems. At first, you might need to refrain from doing things like heavy lifting, extended sitting, or strenuous exercise that could put a strain on the surgical region.

To enhance circulation and avoid blood clots, early ambulation—or brief walks—is frequently advised. Regaining strength and mobility requires gradually increasing your degree of activity as tolerated. Depending on how well you are recovering, your doctor will give you advice on whether it is safe to go back to your regular activities, such as driving or going back to work.

It's common to feel a little tired and have some little pain when exercising in the first few weeks following surgery. Pay attention to your body.

CHAPTER FIVE

MANAGING COMPLICATIONS

Typical Complications and How to Handle Them

Although problems after hemorrhoidectomy are rare, it's nevertheless vital to be aware of the possibility of them occurring. One of the most prevalent problems is pain, which is typically easily treated with prescription painkillers. In situations where pain is worse than anticipated, your doctor may modify your pain management plan or suggest extra methods to relieve discomfort, such as topical therapies or sitz baths.

Bleeding is yet another possible consequence. While some bleeding is common in the first few days following surgery, severe bleeding or bleeding that lasts longer than a few days needs to be immediately reported to your physician. Care may include close observation, a potential follow-up visit to the surgical site to locate the bleeding source, and in extreme circumstances, another surgery.

With any surgical procedure, infection is a potential issue. Increased redness, swelling, warmth, or a pus-like discharge coming from the surgical site are all indicators of infection. Proper wound care practices, such as keeping the region clean and dry, carefully adhering to post-operative instructions, and taking prescription antibiotics as advised by your doctor, are examples of preventive strategies.

Complications including blood clots or trouble urinating could happen seldom. Because of the restricted movement following surgery, deep vein thrombosis, or blood clots, may form in the legs' veins. To reduce this risk, your healthcare team could advise early mobilization, leg exercises, and even blood thinner prescriptions. Urinary retention, or difficulty urinating, may necessitate a temporary urinary catheterization until normal bladder function is restored.

Signs Of Infection And Preventive Actions

After a hemorrhoidectomy, infection is a serious worry, though it is uncommon if treated properly. Increased pain, swelling, redness, warmth, or the appearance of pus-like discharge coming from the surgical site are all indicators of infection. It's critical to carefully adhere to your healthcare provider's wound care guidelines. This usually entails changing dressings as directed, keeping the area dry and clean, and avoiding needless contact or infection.

Your doctor might prophylactically give antibiotics to avoid infection, particularly if you have specific risk factors or the surgery was extensive. To stop bacterial development and lower the chance of infection, it's imperative to take these antibiotics exactly as directed. Further reducing the risk of infection is upholding proper hygiene habits, such as washing hands both before and after tending to the surgery site.

Managing Hemorrhage Following Surgery

Following a hemorrhoidectomy, some bleeding is typical and expected. It is imperative to swiftly seek medical help if the bleeding becomes significant or continues longer than what your healthcare practitioner has recommended as typical. Using clean gauze or a cloth to provide pressure to the area and avoiding activities like heavy lifting or straining during bowel movements could be part of the initial therapy.

To help with clotting and healing, your doctor might advise keeping the area clean and dry, changing dressings frequently, and possibly applying topical treatments or medicated pads. Your healthcare professional may need to perform additional evaluation in situations of severe or ongoing bleeding to identify the reason and the best course of action, which may involve returning to the surgical site for additional intervention.

Managing The Retention Of Urine

Sometimes, swelling or irritation of the nerves around the bladder following a hemorrhoidectomy causes urinary retention or difficulty peeing. The inability to completely or at all empty the bladder may arise from this. Tell your healthcare practitioner right away if you have ongoing pain or find it difficult to urinate within the anticipated time after surgery.

To treat urinary retention, it may be necessary to use a urinary catheter to temporarily empty the bladder until regular urination occurs again. Based on your unique recovery, your doctor will closely evaluate your condition and decide how long to utilize the catheter. To assist with regular urination, they could also suggest supporting measures like medicine to help relax the muscles in the bladder.

Long-Term Issues And Their Resolutions

Chronic discomfort, fecal incontinence, or hemorrhoidal recurrence are rare but possible long-term consequences after a hemorrhoidectomy. To enhance quality of life, chronic pain may necessitate continuing pain management techniques like medication or physical therapy.

Despite being uncommon, fecal incontinence may require specific care depending on how severe it is. This care may include diet adjustments, pelvic floor exercises, or in certain situations, surgery to fix the problem.

Even after surgery, hemorrhoids can recur. Your healthcare physician can suggest cautious measures like dietary adjustments, increased fiber consumption, or topical therapies if symptoms recur over time. If conservative therapies fail, a repeat hemorrhoidectomy or other procedures might be considered in certain circumstances.

You and your healthcare provider can take proactive measures to manage your recovery and general health following a hemorrhoidectomy by being aware of these potential long-term consequences and the therapies associated with them.

To address any issues and maximize your long-term outcomes, you must schedule regular follow-up sessions and maintain open contact with your medical team.

CHAPTER SIX

END RESULTS AND POST-ITEMS

Keeping An Eye Out For Hemorrhoids To Recur

Following a hemorrhoidectomy, it is imperative to keep an eye out for any indications of recurrence. Although this procedure successfully removes hemorrhoids that are already present, new ones may eventually form. Patients should be aware that symptoms like discomfort, itching, or bleeding in the anal region could be signs of a recurrence. Patients should gently examine the area regularly to look for any odd changes. This is known as self-examination. Any worries should be brought up right away with a healthcare professional.

Hemorrhoids might return occasionally due to lifestyle factors like straining during bowel movements, chronic constipation, or a sedentary lifestyle. Thus, consuming a well-balanced, high-fiber diet, drinking plenty of water, and exercising frequently can all help lower the chance of recurrence. These dietary changes assist both the long-term efficacy of the hemorrhoidectomy and general digestive health.

Long-Term Modifications To Lifestyle To Avoid Recurrence

Making some lifestyle adjustments is quite helpful in preventing hemorrhoids from returning after surgery. First off, eating a high-fiber diet softens stools and lessens the need for straining when having a bowel movement. Including an abundance of fruits, veggies, whole grains, and legumes in each meal will help you achieve this. A high-fiber diet is enhanced by enough water, which keeps feces soft and easy to pass.

Regular physical exercise is another crucial element of post-hemorrhoidectomy therapy. Exercise can stop new hemorrhoids from forming by enhancing circulation and bowel function. Easy exercises like yoga, swimming, or walking might be especially beneficial. It's also advisable to avoid standing or sitting for extended periods as this can lead to increased pressure on the rectal veins.

Frequent Follow-Up Plans

After a hemorrhoidectomy, patients usually have follow-up appointments regularly with their physician. These consultations have multiple functions, such as tracking the patient's healing process, evaluating potential problems, and addressing any worries they may have. The medical professional may examine the anal region physically during these visits and talk about any changes in symptoms or general health.

The frequency of follow-up appointments varies based on the particular surgical method utilized as well as the patient's rate of recovery. First appointments can usually be made a few weeks after surgery, with future visits spaced out over several months. These follow-up appointments are crucial to confirming that the patient's recovery is going according to plan and that the surgical site heals appropriately.

Effect On Life Quality

A hemorrhoidectomy can have a major effect on a person's quality of life, especially if they had hemorrhoids before surgery and were in constant pain, bleeding, or discomfort. After the operation, many patients report a significant improvement in their general state of well-being. Relieving symptoms like bleeding, itching, and soreness after bowel movements might make one feel more at ease and confident performing everyday tasks.

Moreover, it is important to recognize the psychological effects of being free of the bothersome symptoms related to hemorrhoids. A higher quality of life frequently contributes to better mental and emotional health in addition to physical health. In testimonies, patients often express pleasure and satisfaction, emphasizing how the operation has improved their capacity to actively participate in work, social activities, and personal relationships, as well as how it has relieved chronic suffering.

Case Studies And Patient Testimonials

Case studies and patient testimonies offer insightful perspectives into the actual experiences of people who have had a hemorrhoidectomy. These narratives frequently describe the course of events from the onset of symptoms and diagnosis to the choice to have surgery and its consequences. Testimonials generally highlight symptom reduction, enhanced quality of life, and the procedure's overall efficacy in treating hemorrhoidal problems.

Case studies, on the other hand, provide a more clinical viewpoint by describing particular patient characteristics, surgical methods used, and results obtained. They function as teaching resources for patients and healthcare professionals alike, demonstrating the efficacy of hemorrhoidectomy in various contexts. Case studies help to clarify the function of surgical intervention in hemorrhoidal disease management by showing both positive outcomes and possible drawbacks.

In summary, long-term results and follow-up following a hemorrhoidectomy are important components of patient care intended to guarantee the best possible recovery, avoid recurrence, and improve quality of life. People can effectively traverse the post-surgery phase and have long-term relief from hemorrhoidal problems by adhering to good living practices, scheduling regular follow-up consultations, and learning from patient testimonials and case studies.

CHAPTER SEVEN

HEMORRHOID TREATMENTS WITH ANOTHER APPROACH

Synopsis Of Non-Surgical Interventions

When it comes to mild to moderate cases of hemorrhoids, non-surgical remedies are frequently the first to be tried. These methods, which do not require intrusive procedures, concentrate on discomfort relief and inflammation reduction. A popular approach involves making dietary and lifestyle adjustments. Increasing fiber consumption is one of these modifications, as it helps soften stools and lessen straining during bowel motions. To maintain softer stools and avoid constipation, which can exacerbate hemorrhoids, this method also promotes drinking enough water.

The management of hemorrhoid symptoms is significantly aided by over-the-counter drugs. Goods that relieve itching and discomfort include topical creams with hydrocortisone or witch hazel. They function by calming the afflicted area and lowering inflammation. Moreover, oral fiber supplements or stool softeners could be suggested to encourage easier bowel motions and reduce stress.

Herbal therapies are among the extra possibilities provided by alternative medicine. Certain herbs, such as butcher's broom and horse chestnut, are thought to have anti-inflammatory qualities that might lessen hemorrhoidal swelling. These supplements come in a variety of formats, such as teas, ointments, and pills. Some people find that these natural methods relieve their symptoms, albeit their efficacy may differ.

The Efficacy Of Dietary And Lifestyle Modifications

Changing one's diet and way of life is essential for treating hemorrhoids. Increasing dietary fiber from foods like fruits, vegetables, and whole grains helps soften and facilitate the passage of feces, hence lessening discomfort and hemorrhoidal bleeding. By keeping stool soft and avoiding constipation, which is a typical aggravating factor for hemorrhoids, adequate water serves as a complement to fiber consumption.

Frequent exercise has additional advantages. Being physically active enhances circulation and bowel function, which might lessen the chance of hemorrhoids occurring or getting worse. Hemorrhoidal veins can be relieved by promoting good blood flow to the rectal area and avoiding extended periods of sitting or standing.

Taking Over-The-Counter Drugs

Many over-the-counter drugs can be used to treat hemorrhoids. These consist of topical ointments and lotions that reduce swelling, discomfort, and itching. Products with hydrocortisone or witch hazel as active components are frequently used to relieve pain and reduce inflammation. They can quickly relieve acute symptoms and are usually applied immediately to the affected area.

Oral over-the-counter drugs like fiber supplements or stool softeners may be advised in addition to topical therapies. Stool softeners function by hydrating feces, which facilitates passage and lessens effort during bowel motions. Conversely, fiber supplements help keep stools soft and regular, which can reduce pain and stop hemorrhoids from getting worse.

The Function Of Complementary And Alternative Medicine

Hemorrhoids can be managed in several ways with alternative medicine, which frequently emphasizes natural cures and comprehensive care. The alleged anti-inflammatory qualities of herbal medicines like butcher's broom and horse chestnut make them attractive options. These herbs, which come in a variety of forms such as ointments, teas, and capsules, are thought to lessen the pain and swelling brought on by hemorrhoids.

Other complementary and alternative remedies include sitz baths, which include submerging the lower body in warm water to induce relaxation and minimize edema surrounding the anus.

This easy method can temporarily relieve pain and itching-related problems. These alternate methods can be strengthened by lifestyle adjustments including the use of hemorrhoid cushions or pillows to lessen pressure on the rectal region when sitting for extended periods.

Comparative Analysis Of Surgical Results

When deciding between surgery and non-surgical therapies for hemorrhoids, it's critical to evaluate the results and efficacy of each strategy.

To reduce discomfort and stop recurrence, non-surgical treatments emphasize symptom management and lifestyle changes. While many people may find relief with these techniques, compared to surgical procedures, they are typically less invasive and have fewer dangers.

On the other hand, surgical results are usually more conclusive when severe hemorrhoids are involved or when non-surgical treatments have not sufficiently relieved the condition.

Hemorrhoids that are large or persistent and do not respond to conservative treatment can be effectively treated with procedures like hemorrhoidectomy, which involves surgically removing hemorrhoidal tissue.

Surgical methods can provide patients with severe hemorrhoidal problems with a long-term remedy, despite the dangers involved, including pain during recovery and possible consequences.

When comparing various methods, it is important to take into account variables including the intensity of the patient's symptoms, patient preferences, and medical professionals' recommendations.

Because non-surgical treatments have a reduced risk profile and have the potential to ameliorate symptoms, they are frequently chosen initially.

When conservative management methods fail to dramatically improve the quality of life due to hemorrhoids, surgical solutions become even more crucial.

CHAPTER EIGHT

FAQS & FREQUENTLY ASKED QUESTIONS

Taking Care Of Common Patient Myths And Fears

Many patients have misunderstandings and worries while considering a hemorrhoidectomy, which can cause needless anxiety.

A widely held misconception is that hemorrhoid surgery is extremely painful and necessitates a protracted recuperation period. Although some discomfort is normal after surgery, contemporary methods and pain management approaches greatly lessen the severity and length of pain.

The possibility of incontinence following a hemorrhoidectomy is another common concern. But this is very uncommon, particularly when done by a skilled surgeon. Patients frequently worry about the possibility of problems, but these can be reduced by doing comprehensive preoperative assessments and adhering to postoperative care guidelines.

The idea that there is only one method for treating hemorrhoids is another fallacy. In actuality, recommendations for surgery are typically made only after non-surgical techniques, drugs, and dietary modifications have failed as therapies.

This indicates that each patient's decision to have a hemorrhoidectomy is unique and is made after carefully weighing all of their options.

Expectations For Pain And Recovery Time

Many of the anxieties associated with hemorrhoidectomy might be allayed by being aware of the pain and anticipated recovery period.

When recommended medication and appropriate care are received, postoperative pain is typically manageable. Following surgery, patients usually feel the most uncomfortable during the first few days, but by the end of the first week, their condition has significantly improved. Patients typically resume their regular activities in a week or two, however, full healing may require several weeks longer.

Patients are urged to adhere to their surgeon's advice regarding medication, hygiene, and degree of exercise to effectively manage pain. Warm water immersions in the anal region, known as Sitz baths, can offer substantial alleviation and aid in the healing process. To promote easy bowel movements and lessen the strain on the surgical site, patients are also advised to refrain from physically demanding activities and to consume a diet high in fiber.

Surgical Risks And Their Management

Hemorrhoidectomy includes some hazards, much like any surgical surgery, but these are carefully controlled to guarantee patient safety. Bleeding, infection, and anesthesia-related responses are common hazards. Nonetheless, these issues are uncommon and are reduced by careful surgical methods and thorough preoperative evaluations.

Enforcing stringent sterile protocols during surgery and administering antibiotics as needed helps prevent infection. During the surgery, bleeding is managed, and it is closely observed afterward.

It is recommended that patients notify their healthcare physician right away if they have severe bleeding. Risks associated with anesthesia are reduced by careful assessments and supervision by skilled anesthesiologists.

Patients are advised to adhere to all preoperative and postoperative care recommendations, including scheduling follow-up sessions to track their progress, to further minimize hazards.

Cost And Insurance Considerations

For many people, having a hemorrhoidectomy might be a major financial concern, but being aware of insurance benefits and associated costs can help with budgeting. Hemorrhoidectomy is usually covered by health insurance companies, particularly if it is considered medically necessary. However, the plan and the provider may have an impact on the coverage's scope. To confirm coverage information, including deductibles, copayments, and out-of-pocket costs, patients should get in touch with their insurance provider.

Patients should think about possible supplemental expenses including prescription drugs, follow-up visits, and preoperative consultations in addition to insurance.

To prevent unanticipated costs, it is advisable to negotiate these fees with the healthcare practitioner in advance. To aid with cost management, a lot of medical facilities provide payment plans or financial assistance programs. Patients can focus on their recovery and have less financial stress if they are well-informed about these possibilities.

Comprehensive Responses To Commonly Asked Questions

A hemorrhoidectomy: what is it?

A surgical technique known as a hemorrhoidectomy is used to remove severe hemorrhoids that are unresponsive to other forms of treatment. To ease symptoms like discomfort, bleeding, and prolapse, the hemorrhoidal tissue is excised during a procedure that is often done under a general anesthetic.

What is the duration of the surgery?

The duration of the treatment varies between 30 and 60 minutes, contingent on the intricacy and quantity of hemorrhoids to be extracted. Patients should, however, budget more time for the surgical center's postoperative recuperation and preparatory needs.

What kind of recuperation can I anticipate?

Both pain management and wound care are essential components of recovery. Patients should adhere to the dietary, exercise, and pain management recommendations made by their surgeon. While most people can get back to their regular schedules in a week or two, full recovery may take longer.

After surgery, are there any food restrictions?

Yes, to promote gentle bowel movements and lessen the tension on the surgery site, patients are frequently advised to maintain a high-fiber diet. Excessive water consumption is also essential. Patients may be advised to start with soft meals and work their way back to a regular diet as they heal.

What should I do if difficulties arise?

Patients should notify their healthcare practitioner right once any complications, such as heavy bleeding, excruciating pain, or infection symptoms (fever, increased redness, or swelling), appear. Appointments for follow-up are necessary to track the healing process and handle any issues.

Is a hemorrhoidectomy a long-term fix?

Hemorrhoids that have already formed can be successfully removed by hemorrhoidectomy, but new ones can still develop. By eating a balanced diet, drinking plenty of water, and avoiding extended sitting or straining during bowel motions, patients can lower their chance of recurrence. Maintaining a healthy weight and engaging in regular exercise are also essential for preventing hemorrhoids from recurring.

www.ingramcontent.com/pod-product-compliance
Lightning Source LLC
Chambersburg PA
CBHW071840210526
45479CB00001B/227